Super
HIGH
INTENSITY
INTERCOURSE
TRAINING

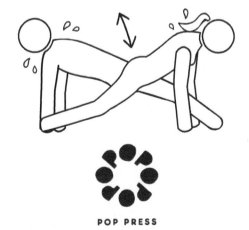

POP PRESS

I'm Joe Dicks, the very personal trainer to those who want to get fit while they get jiggy, and this is the **SHIIT – Super High Intensity Intercourse Training**.

Many of you will have already completed my bestselling **phase 1** of the training programme – **High Intensity Intercourse Training** – and I hope you're ready to crank things up and really feel the burn.

Take your workout to the next level with some powerful special equipment and penetrating exercises that will improve your balance, core strength and flexibility, as well as burn that fat. Let's get set, and sweat.

It's time to get fit or cum trying.

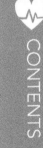

CONTENTS

'When the going gets tough, the tough get shagging.'

If you want to get hench, offer a seat on your firm **bench**.

60 Seconds Pumping
20 Seconds Rest

Difficulty

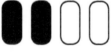

Challenging

Intensity

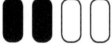

Level 2

CORE

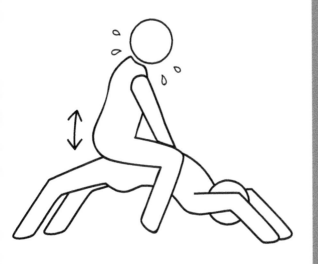

CORE

A boner-fide route to a **scorching-hot** bod.

60 Seconds Pumping
20 Seconds Rest

Difficulty

Expert

Intensity

Level 4

CORE

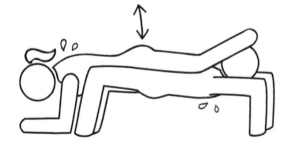

Not everyone's cup of tea/warm piss, but for your pelvic floor it's **bliss**.

5 Seconds of Release
10 Seconds Tensing
Holding Back Flow

Difficulty

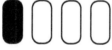

Easy Pee-sy

Intensity

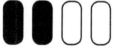

Level 2

CORE

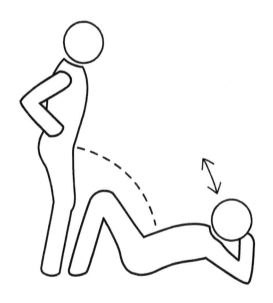

CORE

When the supports are strong, this **bridge** just can't go wrong.

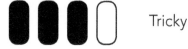

60 Seconds Pumping
20 Seconds Rest

Difficulty

Tricky

Intensity

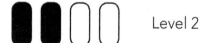

Level 2

CORE

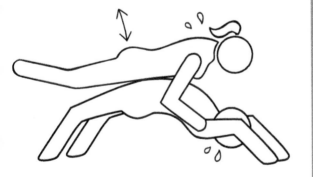

Go super strong for super long to do justice to the **Supergirl**.

60 Seconds Pumping
20 Seconds Rest

Difficulty

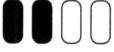

Challenging

Intensity

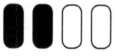

Level 2

CORE

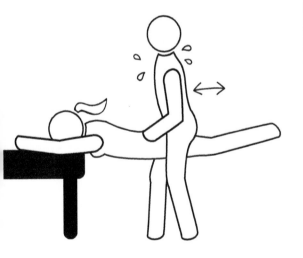

CORE

Be careful – you could get lost in this **three-way**!

 60 Seconds Pumping
20 Seconds Rest

Difficulty

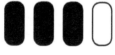 Tricky

Intensity

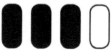 Level 3

CORE

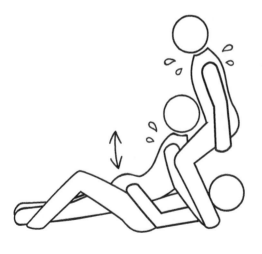

CORE

Keep your eyes on the prize with these abdominal **crunches**.

20 Stomach Crunches while She Pumps
20 Seconds Rest

Difficulty

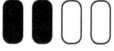

Challenging

Intensity

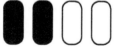

Level 2

CORE

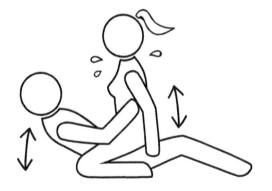

Two's company, three's a crowd – and four's a **Square Meal**, where no one gets left out.

60 Seconds Fun
20 Seconds Rest

Difficulty

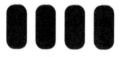

Expert

Intensity

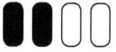

Level 2

CORE

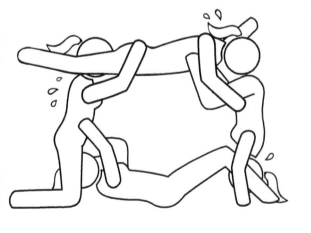

Why not put on a show for that full-body cardio warm-up? Before holding that pose and indulging in **Pole Pleasure**.

60 Seconds Fun
20 Seconds Rest

Difficulty

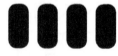

Expert

Intensity

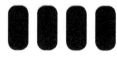

Level 4

Special Equipment Needed
Vertical Pole

CORE

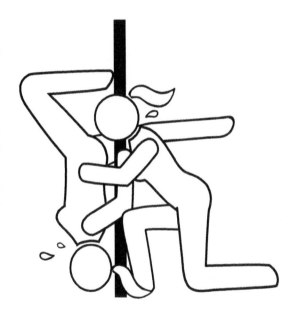

CORE

Get caught between two **desirable** options and plump for both. Have your cock and eat it, in other words.

60 Seconds of Pumping
20 Seconds Rest

Difficulty

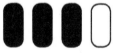

Tricky

Intensity

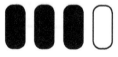

Level 3

CORE

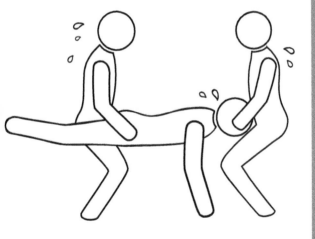

CORE

'Don't tell me the sky's the limit when I've been to heaven and back in the sack.'

Don't let go of her back
or you might feel a sharp
CRACK!

60 Seconds Pumping
20 Seconds Rest

Difficulty

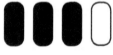

Tricky

Intensity

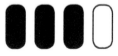

Level 3

THE HOLD STEADY

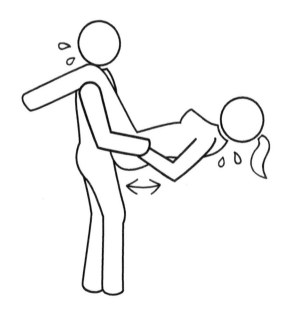

BACK

Arch your back and get fit in the sack.

60 Seconds Pumping
20 Seconds Rest

Difficulty

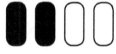

Challenging

Intensity

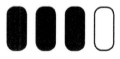

Level 3

BACK

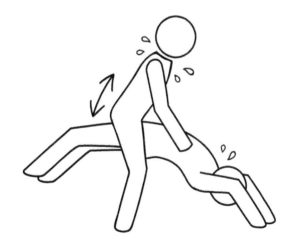

BACK

Shoulder this burden and the **pay-off** is certain.

60 Seconds Fun
20 Seconds Rest

Difficulty

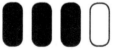

Tricky

Intensity

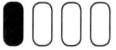

Level 1

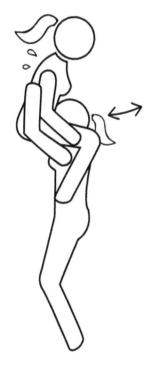

BACK

Back-breaking work – but enjoy the **ride**.

60 Seconds Pumping
20 Seconds Rest

Difficulty

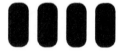

Expert

Intensity

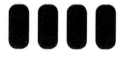

Level 4

BACK

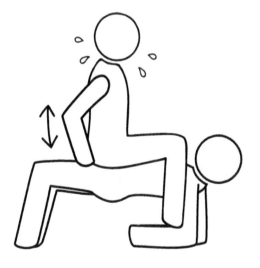

Say no to a life of leisure with this **double-headed** pleasure.

 60 Seconds Pleasure
20 Seconds Rest

Difficulty

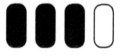 Tricky

Intensity

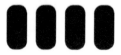 Level 4

BACK

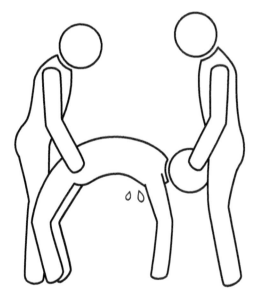

Take your **69** vertical and feel the burn.

 60 Seconds Pumping
20 Seconds Rest

Difficulty

 Expert

Intensity

 Level 3

BACK

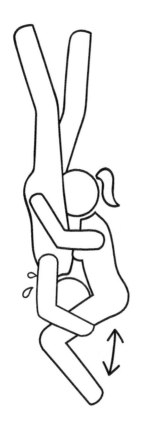

BACK

It's inside you!
Oh yes – **YES, YES!** – it is.

60 Seconds Pumping
20 Seconds Rest

Difficulty

Expert

Intensity

Level 4

BACK

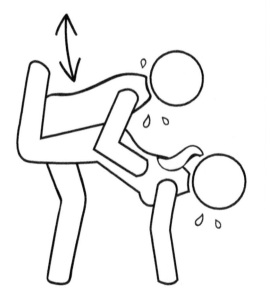

BACK

You'll need to be limber and thorough to **Plough** this particular **Furrow**.

60 Seconds Fun
20 Seconds Rest

Difficulty

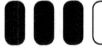

Tricky

Intensity

Level 3

BACK

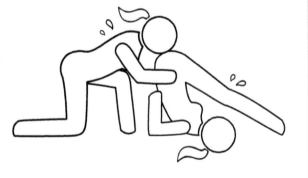

BACK

Any sexual persuasion can enjoy this position – so long as they remember to keep their body as **Straight as an Arrow**.

60 Seconds Pumping
20 Seconds Rest

Difficulty

Expert

Intensity

Level 4

BACK

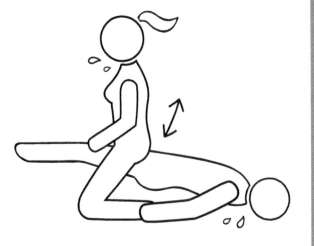

BACK

'Anything worth doing is going to be HARD.'

 LEGS

Squat, thrust, squat, thrust
… find your rhythm and the rewards are just.

10 Squats while Pumping
10 Seconds Pure Pumping
(and repeat)

Difficulty

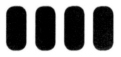

Expert

Intensity

Level 3

LEGS

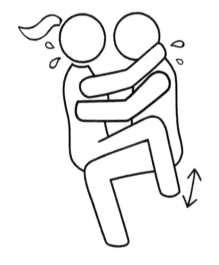

Bedroom gymnastics at their finest – lift her like a barbell as she does the splits, and don't forget to **lick**!

60 Seconds Pumping
20 Seconds Rest

Difficulty

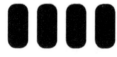

Expert

Intensity

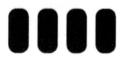

Level 4

LEGS

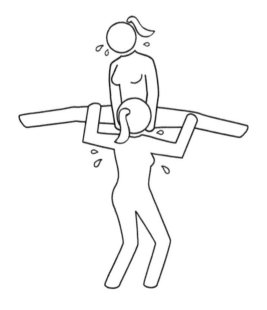

Everyone's a winner with this full-body **sexercise** for two.

60 Seconds Pumping
20 Seconds Rest

Difficulty

Tricky

Intensity

Level 3

LEGS

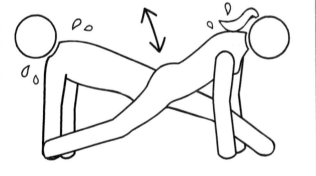

Gently down the stream –
merrily, merrily, merrily, this
will make you **scream**!

 60 Seconds Pumping
20 Seconds Rest

Difficulty

 Tricky

Intensity

 Level 3

LEGS

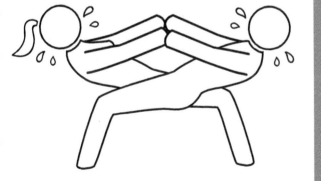

LEGS

Cum together when the **Starter's Gun** fires.

60 Seconds Pumping
20 Seconds Rest

Difficulty

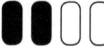

Challenging

Intensity

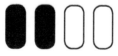

Level 2

LEGS

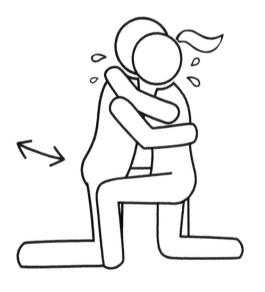

LEGS

Supplicate and fornicate
before the gods of
sexual fitness.

60 Seconds Pumping
20 Seconds Rest

Difficulty

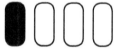

Beginner Level

Intensity

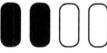

Level 2

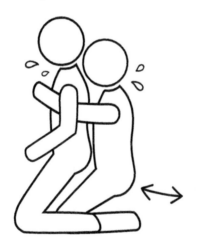

Talk is cheap – **Split the Difference** and get nice and deep.

 60 Seconds Pumping
20 Seconds Rest

Difficulty

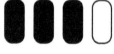 Tricky

Intensity

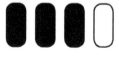 Level 3

LEGS

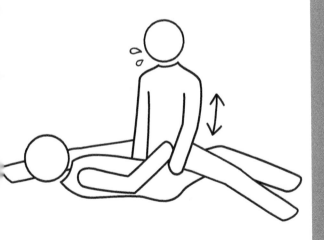

LEGS

No need to make a wish on this **Shooting Star** – it's already cum true.

60 Seconds Fun
20 Seconds Rest

Difficulty

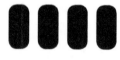

Expert

Intensity

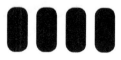

Level 4

LEGS

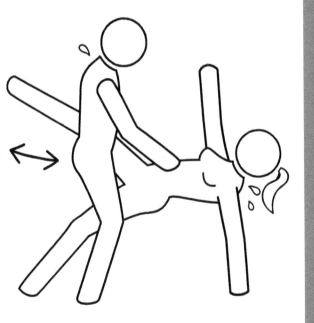

LEGS

No **monkeying around** – set the bar high so orgasms abound.

60 Seconds Pumping
20 Seconds Rest

Difficulty

Tricky

Intensity

Level 4

Special Equipment Needed
Pull-up Bar

LEGS

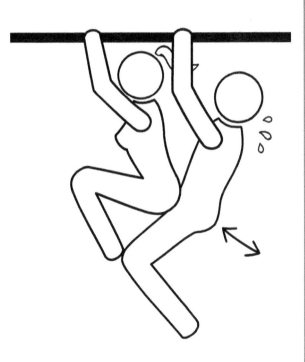

LEGS

'Eye of the tiger
– sex drive of
the rabbit.'

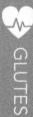

GLUTES

If it's a tight body you want,
it's time to **Tuck It In**.

60 Seconds Pumping
20 Seconds Rest

Difficulty

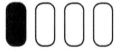

Beginner Level

Intensity

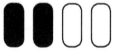

Level 2

GLUTES

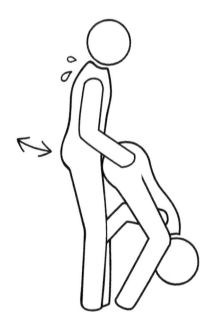

GLUTES

Ride this rocket into space and you're sure to see stars.

 60 Seconds Pumping
20 Seconds Rest

Difficulty

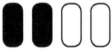 Challenging

Intensity

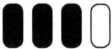 Level 3

GLUTES

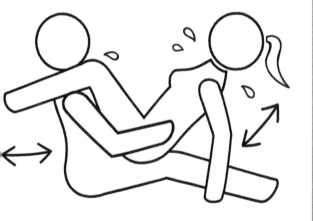

GLUTES

Hold that pose even as she **blows**.

60 Seconds Pumping
20 Seconds Rest

Difficulty

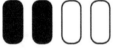

Challenging

Intensity

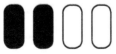

Level 2

GLUTES

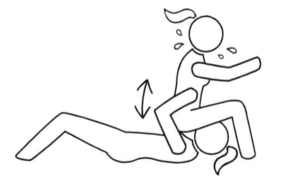

No need for a **protractor** – just get on and shaft her!

60 Seconds Pumping
20 Seconds Rest

Difficulty

Challenging

Intensity

Level 3

Special Equipment Needed
Yoga Harness

GLUTES

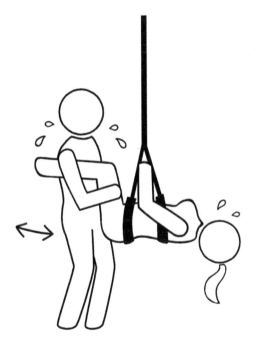

GLUTES

With this on your lap you won't want to **change channels**.

60 Seconds Pumping
20 Seconds Rest

Difficulty

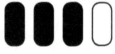

Tricky

Intensity

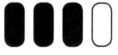

Level 3

GLUTES

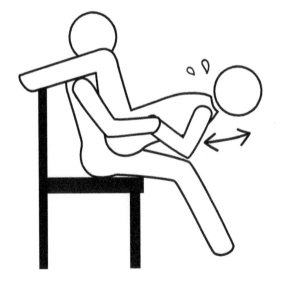

GLUTES

Drive carefully and considerately over this **Hump in the Road** – and your body will thank you for it afterwards.

 60 Seconds Humping
20 Seconds Rest

Difficulty

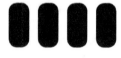 Expert

Intensity

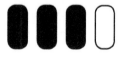 Level 3

GLUTES

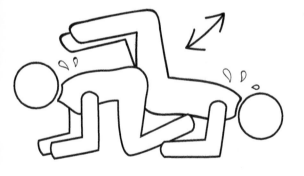

GLUTES

Make like a backwards roll
as you slide on to his **pole**.

60 Seconds Pumping
20 Seconds Rest

Difficulty

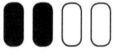

Challenging

Intensity

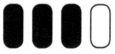

Level 3

ROLY-POLY

GLUTES

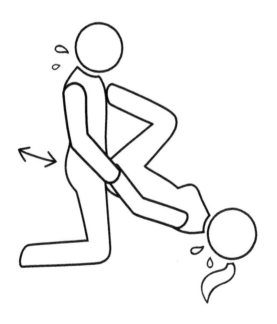

GLUTES

Screw nice and tight if you want your glutes to feel just right.

60 Seconds Pumping
20 Seconds Rest

Difficulty

Tricky

Intensity

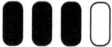

Level 3

GLUTES

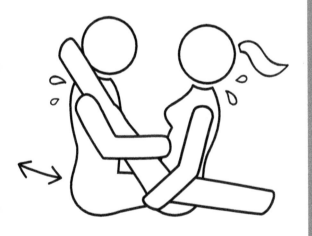

GLUTES

'On good days, shag. On bad days, shag harder.'

Forget your **S&M** hang-ups – put your arm into it and bulge up your biceps.

60 Seconds Pleasure and Battle Rope Waves
20 Seconds Rest and Change Hands

Difficulty

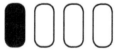

Beginner Level

Intensity

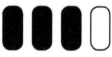

Level 3

Special Equipment Needed
Battle Rope

ARMS

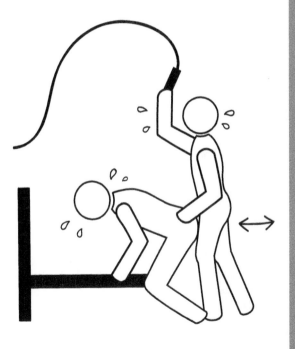

ARMS

Forget the **Pirate's Code** – shag this plank.

60 Seconds Pumping
20 Seconds Rest

Difficulty

Challenging

Intensity

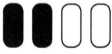

Level 2

ARMS

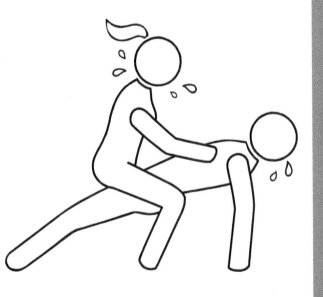

ARMS

Give this **tongue twister** a go and bend your body to your will.

60 Seconds Fun
20 Seconds Rest

Difficulty

Challenging

Intensity

Level 3

ARMS

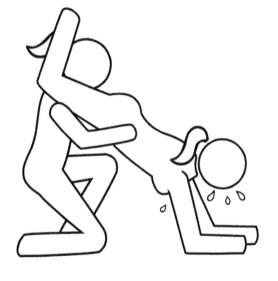

ARMS

Bodyweight exercises get a whole lot more interesting with another **hot bod** on board.

60 Seconds Pumping
20 Seconds Rest

Difficulty

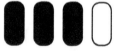

Tricky

Intensity

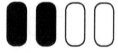

Level 2

Special Equipment Needed
TRX Trainer

COCKY CALISTHENICS

ARMS

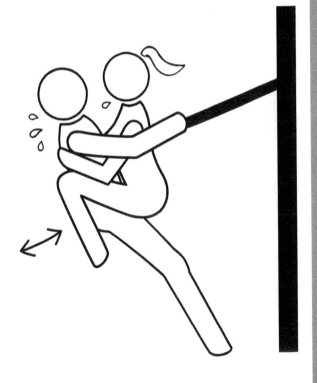

ARMS

Find your inner Patrick Swayze – and lift your partner into a **sexual haze**.

Hold and Pleasure for 60 Seconds
20 Seconds Rest

Difficulty

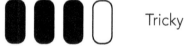

Tricky

Intensity

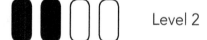

Level 2

DIRTY, DIRTY DANCING

ARMS

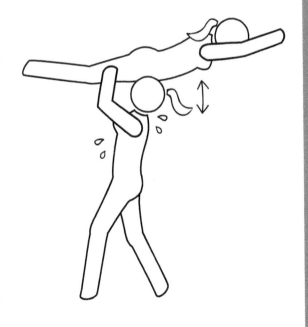

The **rush** you'll get from this won't just be the blood to your head.

 60 Seconds Fun
20 Seconds Rest

Difficulty

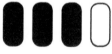 Tricky

Intensity

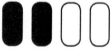 Level 2

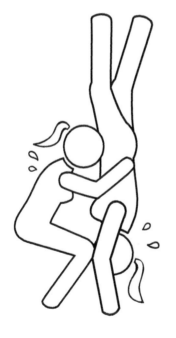

ARMS

Who needs the gym when you can get fit licking a **rim**.

 20 Seconds Fun
20 Seconds Rest

Difficulty

 Tricky

Intensity

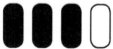 Level 3

ARMS

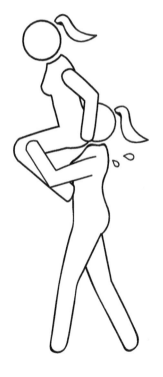

ARMS

Pull-ups are for wimps – you need to get your **pecker up**.

20 Pull-Ups
20 Seconds Rest

Difficulty

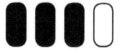

Tricky

Intensity

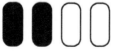

Level 2

Special Equipment Needed
Pull-up Bar

ARMS

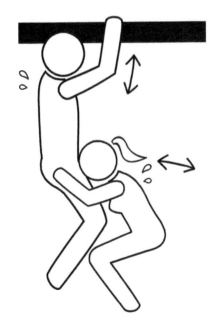

ARMS

Take your **dawg** for walkies for an extra-intense work-out.

 60 Seconds Pumping
20 Seconds Rest

Difficulty

 Challenging

Intensity

 Level 2

ARMS

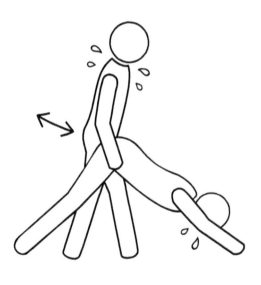

ARMS

Screw her **lotus** but don't lose focus!

60 Seconds Pumping
20 Seconds Rest

Difficulty

Tricky

Intensity

Level 3

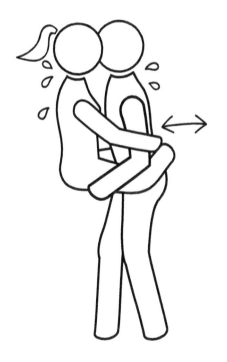

ARMS

A press-up isn't **hardcore** till it's done with your knuckles – and someone's mouth between your legs.

20 Press-ups
20 Seconds Rest

Difficulty

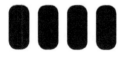

Expert

Intensity

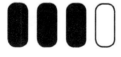

Level 3

ARMS

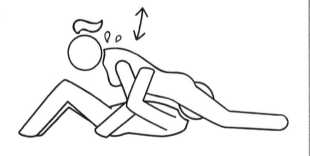

'It's tough at the top (and it isn't always a breeze on the bottom).'

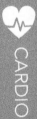

Hold on to that headboard and get your **heart rate** up!

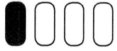

60 Seconds Pumping
20 Seconds Rest

Difficulty

Beginner Level

Intensity

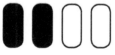

Level 2

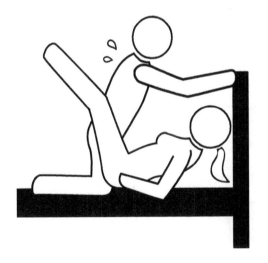

An **on-the-go** exercise that works just as well in a public toilet as it does a secluded alleyway.

 60 Seconds Pumping
20 Seconds Rest

Difficulty

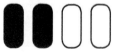 Beginner Level

Intensity

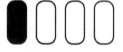 Level 2

KNEE TREMBLER

CARDIO

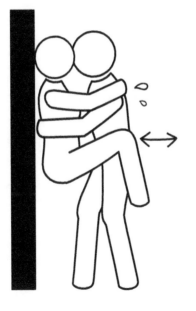

Up the apples and pears ... forget the lift and **get at it** on the stairs.

60 Seconds Pumping
20 Seconds Rest

Difficulty

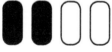

Beginner Level

Intensity

Level 2

CARDIO

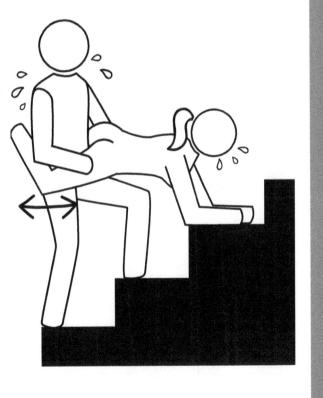

There's more than one way to be a swinger – and make the body of your dreams a very possible **mission**.

60 Seconds Pumping
20 Seconds Rest

Difficulty

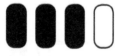

Tricky

Intensity

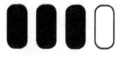

Level 3

Special Equipment Needed
Yoga Harness

CARDIO

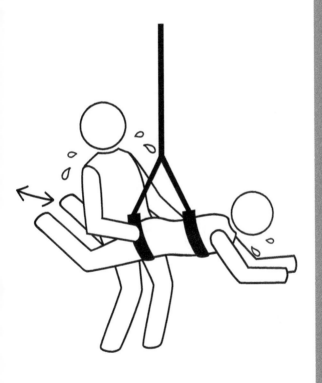

CARDIO

Giddy-up! Make him weak at the knees as you **jockey** for perfect position in this pose.

 60 Seconds Pumping
20 Seconds Rest

Difficulty

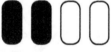 Challenging

Intensity

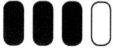 Level 3

CARDIO

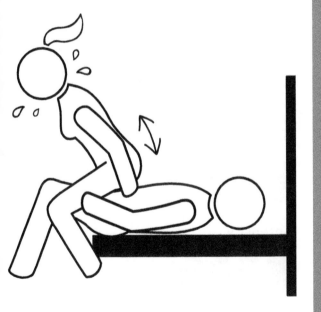

CARDIO

One for the **home gym** – and a sure-fire way to stay slim. (Please wipe down the equipment after use.)

60 Seconds Pumping
20 Seconds Rest

Difficulty

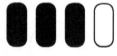

Tricky

Intensity

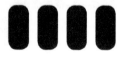

Level 4

Special Equipment Needed
Cross Trainer

CROSS-TRAIN HURRICANE

CARDIO

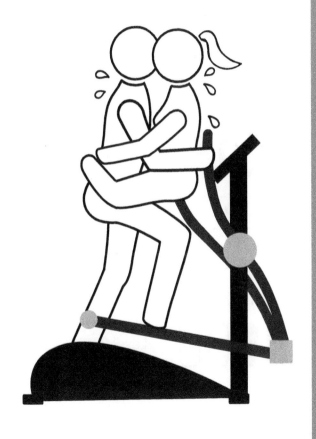

Make this much-maligned position work for you in a punishing cardio **shagathon**.

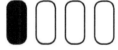

60 Seconds Pumping
20 Seconds Rest

Difficulty

Beginner Level

Intensity

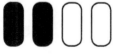

Level 2

MISSIONARY ZEAL

CARDIO

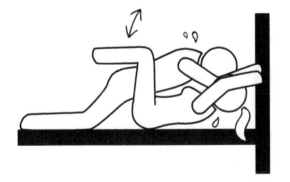

Kung-fu fornication will get the blood pumping – as well as other bodily fluids.

60 Seconds Pumping
20 Seconds Rest

Difficulty

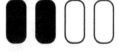

Challenging

Intensity

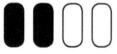

Level 2

CARDIO

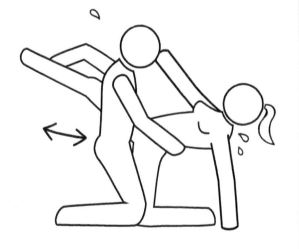

Pimp your doggy style and get airborne – just remember nice and gently when it comes time to '**Down, boy!**'

60 Seconds Pumping
20 Seconds Rest

Difficulty

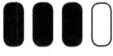

Tricky

Intensity

Level 3

CARDIO

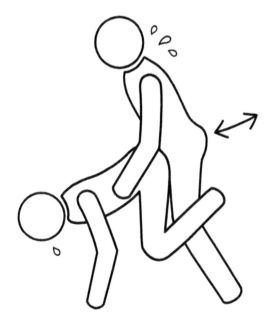

5 7 9 10 8 6 4

Pop Press, an imprint of Ebury Publishing,
20 Vauxhall Bridge Road,
London SW1V 2SA

Pop Press is part of the Penguin Random House group of companies
whose addresses can be found at global.penguinrandomhouse.com

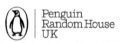

Copyright © Pop Press 2020

First published in the United Kingdom by Pop Press in 2020

www.penguin.co.uk

A CIP catalogue record for this book is available from the
British Library

ISBN 9781529107159

Design by Emily Snape
Joe Dicks would like to thank Steve Burdett
for translating his actions into words.
Project management by whitefox
Printed and bound in Great Britain by Clays Ltd, Elcograf S.p.A.

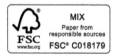